I0419791

Type 2 Diabetes

Smallest book with Everything you need to know

Updated 2nd Edition

Dr. Shahriar Mostafa

MBBS, MPH

Copyright 2016 Dr. Shahriar Mostafa

This ebook is licensed for your personal enjoyment only. This ebook may not be re-sold or given away to other people. Thank you for respecting the hard work of this author.

☐

Preface

Our life has become busier than ever. Living in the age of information, we are connected all the time. Now time is the most valuable thing in our life. On Type 2 Diabetes you can find a thousand websites with million pages. You will also find many books with hundreds of pages. From this ocean of information what you urgently need is hard to find. And it's time-consuming.

This book is small, and you do not have to read this book from page one to the end. You can start anywhere and slowly finish it. Use the table of contents to find the topic of your interest and start from there.

You can finish this book in just 1 hour. In 1 hour, you will have all necessary information on Type 2 Diabetes. This book will give the confidence, hope, and information to live a normal, happy life with Type 2 Diabetes.

This book is the best choice as a gift to your friends, coworkers or Family who has Type 2 Diabetes. Or recently diagnosed with Type 2 Diabetes. This gift will show that you care.

⁇

Table of Contents

Notes

This book is not a prescription from a doctor. Do not change, increase, start or skip any ongoing treatment without consulting your physician.

Please send an email to dr.shahriar@doctor.com. With Type 2 in the subject line, I will email you every update/edition of this book (eBook only) completely free.

Feel free to Email any question, suggestion or mistake to dr.shahriar@doctor.com I will answer your questions.

Without your review, I can't reach others. I request you to write a review if you like or dislike this book. I will mention your review in future editions of this book.

⁇

Introduction

As soon as you learn that you have Type 2 Diabetes, you become terrified. What happens in Type 2 Diabetes? What to do to cure it? How to control it? What's causing it? Why did it happen to me? Thousand and thousand questions pop up in your mind. You become confused, afraid and angry.

But you don't have to be confused or afraid. You are not alone. Diabetes is a common disease. About 350 million people worldwide have diabetes. It is easy to control. It does not keep you from anything the life has to offer. But there is a catch; you have to manage Type 2 Diabetes all your life.

Diabetes is like a shadow of you. Like a shadow, it will always be with you. When controlled like a shadow you will forget even it is present. And in not so distant future, you will be cured of Type 2 Diabetes.

Emotional Issues and Self-Esteem.

Diabetic patients may develop some emotional issues. They tend to develop low self-esteem. The patient feels as if he must be a bad person or have done something wrong to stuck with such a disease. Patients sometimes develop the idea that diabetes makes them less handsome or cute or lower IQ than their friends.

Patients may blame themselves for the disease.

Patients may think diabetes damages your brain and feel inferior. There is a constant fear of complication. The special diets, medication, and blood glucose monitoring are emotionally demanding.

Emotional issues should be treated by counseling and support from family and friends. Professional advice helps to gain self-esteem, reduce depression.

Celebrities with Diabetes

Diabetes does not keep you away from success in your life. You need to believe that. Following are some celebrities with diabetes, it shows if you control your diabetes, there is no problem getting what you want in life.

Halle Berry - Diabetes didn't stop her from appearing as the super-powered mutant Storm in the X-Men movies.

Nick Jonas - This 14-year-old star of the pop rock band the Jonas Brothers were diagnosed with type 1 diabetes in 2007.

Adam Morrison - Diagnosed with type 1 diabetes at age 14, Adam worked hard and made it all the way to the NBA where he plays basketball for the Charlotte Bobcats.

Gary Hall - This Olympic athlete didn't let diabetes stop him from earning a gold medal in swimming.

Elliott Yamin - After being diagnosed with diabetes at age 16, he went on to become one of the top singers on American Idol in 2006.

Vanessa Williams - Not only was Vanessa the first African-American Miss America, but she also has diabetes.

Doug Burns - Mr. Universe doesn't let his diabetes stop him from being an award-winning bodybuilder.

Jackie Robinson - The first black baseball player in the major leagues had diabetes.

Anne Rice - The famous vampire novel writer has diabetes.

George Lucas - The creator of the Star Wars saga is a very mild type 2 diabetic.

Chris Dudley - Before Adam Morrison, Chris Dudley played in the NBA with type 1 diabetes.

Bret Michaels - The lead singer of Poison was diagnosed with diabetes at age six.

Bill and John Davidson - The big bosses at Harley Davidson Motorcycles have diabetes.

Mikhail Gorbachev - The former leader of the Soviet Union has diabetes.

Johnny Cash - The famous country musician was a diabetic.

Elvis Presley - The former king of rock 'n roll had diabetes.

Sharon Stone - Halle's Cat Woman co-star also has diabetes.

Thomas Edison - The inventor of the light bulb had diabetes.

HG Wells - The famed science-fiction author had diabetes.

Nicole Johnson - 1999's Miss America has diabetes.

Kendall Simmons - Busting heads on offense for the Pittsburgh Steelers keeps this diabetic athlete busy."

The list of Successful people and celebrities with diabetes is a long one. Here I have given a small fraction. These peoples show you that diabetes (when controlled) does not get in your way to success. These achievements give you the confidence to deal with Type 2 Diabetes.

What is the condition of Diabetes worldwide?

"About 350 million people worldwide have diabetes. A forecast from world health organization(WHO) Predicts, this number likely to double or more in the next 20 years."

"In 2012, an estimated 1.5 million deaths caused by diabetes. More than 80% of diabetes deaths occur in low- and middle-income countries."

"In 2014 Diabetes worldwide estimated to be 9% among adults aged 18+ years".

"WHO projects that diabetes will be the 7th leading cause of death by the year 2030".

What is Blood sugar or Blood Glucose?

To understand diabetes; first, we have to know what blood sugar is? Where is it coming from? The food we eat contains many substances. After eating, food is broken down into a simple form that our body can use. When food is broken into a simple form, we get three primary substances. Glucose or Sugar from Carbohydrate (rice, pasta, bread, etc.). Fat from oil, butter etc. Protein from meat, milk egg etc.

For diabetes, the carbohydrate or sugar part is important.

The journey of carbohydrate within our body.

Carbohydrate starts its transformation from our mouth to stomach and intestine. Inside our gut food is mashed. Mixed with enzymes and acid and broken down into simple sugar (glucose).

Glucose is the fuel used by our body to do everything we do and keep us alive. Sugar absorbed into the blood as glucose (a primary type of sugar). Body delivers this glucose carried by the blood to every cell of our body.

But glucose can't get inside a cell straight from the blood. For glucose to get inside our cells from blood, we need insulin. Insulin works as a key for glucose to get inside the cells of our body.

What is diabetes?

Insulin is made in our body by an organ called pancreas. If pancreas could not produce insulin in adequate quantity. Or if your cells do not unlock its doors with insulin (insulin resistance). Glucose stays in the blood. This increased glucose level in the blood or hyperglycemia is the condition we call Diabetes.

What happens in Type 2 Diabetes?

Type 2 diabetes develops over a long period (years). People with type 2 diabetes make insulin, but their cells don't use it as well as they should. It is called insulin resistance. In insulin resistance, insulin becomes increasingly ineffective at managing the blood glucose levels.

To correct this blood glucose level pancreas makes more insulin to try to get glucose into the cells. But eventually it can't keep up, and the sugar builds up in your blood.

Usually, a combination of things causes type 2 diabetes, including:

• Genes. Scientists have found different bits of DNA that affect how your body makes insulin.

• Extra weight. Being overweight or obese can cause insulin resistance, especially if you carry your extra pounds around the middle. Now type 2 diabetes affects kids and teens as well as adults, mainly because of childhood obesity.

• Metabolic syndrome. People with insulin resistance often have a group of conditions including high blood glucose, extra fat around the waist, high blood pressure, and high cholesterol and triglycerides.

• Glucose from your liver. When your blood sugar is low, your liver makes and sends out glucose to keep body's functionality active. After you eat, your blood sugar goes up, and usually, the liver will slow down and store its glucose for later. But some people's liver doesn't stop making glucose. They keep cranking out sugar.

Factors causing Type 2 Diabetes?

Type 2 diabetes has a genetic disposition Diabetes runs in the family, if you have a family member with diabetes, most likely you have a genetic disposition to have diabetes. You inherit a predisposition to diabetes, and then you need a triggering event to develop diabetes. Some things in your environment can work as a trigger.

Although there is a strong genetic predisposition, the risk is significantly increased when associated with lifestyle factors such as high blood pressure, overweight or obesity, insufficient physical activity, poor diet and the classic 'apple shape' body where extra weight is carried around the waist.

There is no single cause of type 2 diabetes; there are well-established risk factors. Some risk factors can be controlled and others you are born with.

You are at a higher risk of getting type 2 diabetes if you:

• have a family history of diabetes

• are older (over 55 years of age) - the risk increases as we age, over 45 years of age and are overweight, have a high blood pressure increase risk of diabetes.

• Are over 35 years of age and are from an Aboriginal or Torres Strait Islander background. Or from Pacific Island, the Indian subcontinent or Chinese increase risk of diabetes.

• A woman who had given birth to a child over 4.5 kgs (9 lbs.), or had gestational diabetes when pregnant, or had a condition known as Polycystic Ovarian Syndrome has increased the risk of developing diabetes.

Risk factors for type 2 diabetes

Four of the main risk factors for developing type 2 diabetes are:

Age – being over the age of 40 (over 25 for South Asian people). This risk may be because people tend to gain weight and exercise less as they get older. However, despite increasing age being a risk factor for type 2 diabetes, over recent years' younger people from all ethnic groups have been developing the condition. It's also becoming more common for children, in some cases as young as seven, to develop type 2 diabetes.

Genetics – having a close relative with diabetes (parent, brother or sister). A child who has a parent with type 2 diabetes has about a one in three chance of also developing it

Weight – You're more likely to develop type 2 diabetes if you're overweight or obese (with a body-mass index (BMI) of 30 or more. In particular, fat around your tummy (abdomen) increases your risk. This is because it releases chemicals that can upset the body's cardiovascular and metabolic systems. With diabetes, this increases your risk of developing some serious conditions, including coronary heart disease, stroke and some types of cancer.

Measuring your waist is a quick way of assessing your diabetes risk. This is a measure of abdominal obesity, which is a particularly high-risk form of obesity. Women have a higher risk of developing type 2 diabetes if their waist measures 80cm (31.5 inches) or more. Asian men with a waist size of 89cm (35 inches) or over have a higher risk, as do white or black men with a waist size of 94cm (37 inches) or over.

Use the BMI calculator to find out if you're a healthy weight for your height.

Exercising regularly and reducing your body weight by about 5% could reduce your risk of getting diabetes by more than 50%.

Ethnicity – being of South Asian, Chinese, African-Caribbean or Black African origin (even if you were born in the UK or any other country). People of South Asian, Chinese, African-Caribbean and black African are more likely to develop type 2 diabetes. Type 2 diabetes is up to six times more common in South Asian communities than in the general UK population, and it's three times more common among people of African and African-Caribbean origin.

People of South Asian and African-Caribbean origin also have an increased risk of developing complications of diabetes, such as heart disease, at a younger age than the rest of the population

Other risks

Your risk of developing type 2 diabetes is also increased if your blood glucose level is higher than normal but not yet high enough to be diagnosed with diabetes. This condition is called "pre-diabetes" – doctors sometimes call it impaired fasting glycemia (IFG) or impaired glucose tolerance (IGT).

Pre-diabetes can progress to type 2 diabetes if you don't take preventative steps, such as making lifestyle changes. These include eating healthily, losing weight (if you're overweight) and taking plenty of regular exercises.

Women who have had gestational diabetes during pregnancy also have a greater risk of developing diabetes in later life.

Symptoms of Type 2 Diabetes?

Symptoms of Type 2 Diabetes are;

- **Increased thirst** - when blood glucose level is high. Our body tries to dilute the high blood glucose with water. To meet this increased water demand body signals our thirst center. So thirst increases.

- **Increased frequency of urination**- In diabetes frequency of urination increases. Diabetic patients have high blood glucose. To lower this blood glucose, the body tries to flush out the extra glucose through urine. That's why increased frequency of urination occurs. Diabetic patients may pass urine for more than 20 times a day.

- • **Increased volume of urine** - in hyperglycemia or high blood glucose. The body tries to remove all excessive glucose through urine. So the amount of urine increases up to 3 liters or more.

Other symptoms are

- Weight loss, even after taking enough food.
- Pain in the abdomen.
- Loss of appetite.
- Nausea and vomiting.
- Fatigue or tiredness
- Blurring of vision
- Mood change
- Irritability

- The patient may develop and present with dehydration, unconsciousness.

- Recurrent episodes of urinary & genital tract infections is a sign of diabetes.

Lab tests for Type 2 Diabetes.

Besides symptoms, some tests are done to confirm Type 2 Diabetes. Your doctor will decide which tests are needed. Some standard tests for Type 2 Diabetes are;

Fasting blood glucose - Done after overnight fasting (No food or drinks for at least 8 hours). You have to give a small amount of blood early in the morning on an empty stomach.

- If the test result shows fasting blood glucose level equal or more than 126 mg/dL (7.0 mmol/L). It is a positive sign of diabetes.

2 hours after 75g glucose - In this test after overnight fasting (No food or drinks for at least 8 hours). On an empty stomach, you have to take 75g glucose dissolved in a glass of water. Then after 2 hours, a small amount of blood taken to measure the glucose level in blood.

- Blood glucose level equal or more than 200 mg/dL (11.1 mmol/L) two hours after 75g glucose. Is positive for Diabetes.

If you have symptoms of diabetes or complications of diabetes your doctor may do a random blood glucose level, which can be done anytime. A small amount of blood taken. Random blood glucose equal or more than 200 mg/dL (11.1 mmol/L) is positive for diabetes. It indicates that your doctor should do other tests to confirm the diagnosis of Type 2 Diabetes.

A test called Hemoglobin A1c is also essential.

HbA1c measure glucose in red blood cells. It shows the average blood glucose level for the last 2 to 3 months. It is also useful for treatment & follow-up of a patient with Diabetes. This test can be done anytime. Empty stomach or just after food. Food has no effect on this test result.

HbA1C level more than 6.5% is positive for diabetes. But if you have anemia, sickle cell anemia or thalassemia the test result can be falsely positive.

The HbA1C test should be performed in a laboratory using a method that is NGSP certified and standardized to the DCCT assay.

Other tests specific for Type 2 Diabetes?

To check other diseases. And to screen out the complications of Type 2 Diabetes following tests are usually done.

- Complete Blood Count with Peripheral Blood Film
- Fasting lipid profile – for vascular damage, heart diastase.
- Liver function test.

- Renal function test – to prevent of diabetic kidney disease (Diabetic Nephropathy).

- Electrocardiogram (ECG) etc.

Monitoring of blood sugar at home.

Monitoring blood glucose level in blood is important. Getting pricked with Lancet or syringe is a painful process. But there is no better effective alternative yet. You cannot guess the blood glucose level without a test. The patient can feel only the low blood glucose level, but even then, he can't feel how low it is.

For Type 2 Diabetes you should check the blood glucose as your doctor advised. Sometimes you may have to check blood glucose level at least three times every day. Before every meal. Once every week, check blood glucose one hour after a meal.

Lab test result for blood glucose is almost same using glucometer at home. Glucometer test from the finger blood may vary only 10% of a lab test.

You must maintain a log with date, time, condition (empty stomach or after food) and blood glucose level. Now there are apps available for iOS, Android, and Windows to easily maintain a diabetes log.

Steps to check blood sugar at home?

Start the task of home blood glucose monitoring with making the meter ready. Insert the strip into the meter. Wash your hand, and you may clean the finger with rubbing alcohol or use soap and water. Prick finger to get one drop of blood. Give the blood on the strip. In a few seconds, the meter will display current blood glucose level.

Do finger prick on the side of the finger where pain sensation is little. If available, use low pain lancet. Use alternate finger every time. If blood does not come after finger prick by the Lancet, a gentle squeeze of the finger will help.

Carefully store glucometer strips. Only 2-hour exposure of strips to air will damage the strip. Blood glucose level from finger prick is better than blood from other sites (heel, ear lobe etc.)

Apps for record keeping of Type 2 Diabetes?

Monitoring and keeping the record of type 1 Diabetes is easy now. There are many apps for iPhone, iPad, Android and Windows. To give you an initial idea of these I have reviewed two apps. You can use these apps or find one of your choices.

Diabetes: M

Designed for smartphones and tablets this application is intended to help people with diabetes to manage better their diabetes and keep it under control. Users can log their values in this diary and maintain the records with them all the time. The application tracks almost all aspects of the diabetes treatment and provides detailed reports, charts, and statistics to share via the email with the supervising physician. It provides

various tools to the diabetics, so they can find the trends in blood glucose levels and allows users to calculate normal and prolonged insulin boluses using it's highly effective, top-notch bolus calculator.

"Diabetes: M" can analyze the values from the imported data from various glucometers and insulin pumps via the exported files from their respective diabetes management software systems.

Supports Android Wear smartwatches. The app is available in Android play store and iTunes store.

mySugr Diabetes Logbook

mySugr Logbook app is a charming diabetes tracker for blood glucose, bolus, basal, food, carbs, meds, pills, weight, a1c and more. It makes your diary useful in everyday life with playful elements and immediate feedback through your diabetes monster! Get motivated and involved in your diabetes therapy, today!

— No. 1 diabetes logbook app in 6 countries

— Most popular diabetes logbook app in the world based on five-star reviews and ratings

— Winner of Germany's "Focus Diabetes" 'Best Apps for People with Diabetes' award

Our motto: We make diabetes suck less!

FEATURES/ADD-ONS:

• Designed for type 1 & type 2 diabetes

• Quick and easy logging (meals, meds, BG's, and more)

• Personalized logging screen (add, remove, and reorder fields)

• Estimated HbA1c - so there are no nastier surprises

• CGM data integration via CSV import (only available in German and English speaking countries)

• Daily, weekly, monthly analysis (and more)

• Exciting challenges for personal therapy goals

You can visit the iTunes store or Google play store, and there are a lot of apps for diabetes. You can download those apps and decide which app works for you.

Medicines used for the treatment of Type 2 Diabetes?

There's no cure for diabetes yet, so treatment aims to keep your blood glucose levels as normal as possible and to control your symptoms, to prevent complications.

Type 2 diabetes usually gets worse over time. Making lifestyle changes, such as adjusting your diet and exercise, may help you control your blood glucose levels at first. But they will not be enough in the long term.

You may eventually need to take medication to help control your blood glucose levels. Initially, this will usually be in the form of tablets, and can sometimes be a combination of more than one type of tablet. It may also include insulin or other medication that you inject.

The decision about which medications are best depends on many factors, including your blood sugar level and any other health problems you have. Your doctor might even combine drugs from different classes to help you control your blood sugar.

Available medicines for the treatment of type 2 diabetes include:

Metformin

 Generally, metformin is the first medication prescribed for type 2 diabetes. It is available as an oral tablet or capsule. It works by improving the sensitivity of your body tissues to insulin so that your body uses insulin more efficiently. It makes your body's cells more responsive to insulin. It also works by reducing the amount of glucose that your liver releases into your bloodstream.

Metformin is recommended for adults with a high risk of developing type 2 diabetes, whose blood glucose is still increasing towards type 2 diabetes, despite making necessary lifestyle changes.

If you're overweight, it's also likely you'll be prescribed metformin. Unlike some other medicines used to treat type 2 diabetes, metformin doesn't cause additional weight gain.

Nausea and diarrhea are possible side effects of metformin. These side effects usually go away as your body gets used to metformin. If metformin and lifestyle changes aren't enough to control your blood sugar level, other oral or injected medications can be added.

Sulfonylureas

Sulfonylureas increase the amount of insulin that's produced by your pancreas. Examples of medications in this class include glyburide, glipizide, and glimepiride.

You may be prescribed sulfonylurea if you can't take metformin, or if you aren't overweight. Alternatively, you may be prescribed sulfonylurea and metformin together if metformin doesn't control blood glucose on its own.

Sulphonylureas can increase the risk of hypoglycemia (low blood sugar) because they increase the amount of insulin in your body. They can also sometimes cause side effects, including weight gain, nausea, and diarrhea.

Meglitinides

These medications work like sulfonylureas by stimulating the pancreas to secrete more insulin. They're faster acting, and the duration of their effect in the body is short. They have a risk of causing low blood sugar (hypoglycemia). Weight gain is a possibility with this class of medications.

Thiazolidinediones

these drugs make the body's tissues more sensitive to insulin. This class of medicines has been linked to weight gain and other more-serious side effects, such as an increased risk of heart failure and fractures. Because of these risks, these medications aren't the first-choice treatment.

Thiazolidinedione medicines (pioglitazone) make your body's cells more sensitive to insulin so that more glucose is taken from your blood.

They're usually used in combination with metformin or sulphonylureas, or both. They may cause weight gain and ankle swelling (edema). You shouldn't take pioglitazone if you have heart failure or a high risk of bone fracture.

Another thiazolidinedione, rosiglitazone, was withdrawn from use in 2010 due to an increased risk of cardiovascular disorders, including heart attack and heart failure.

DPP-4 inhibitors

These medications help reduce blood sugar levels but tend to have a modest effect. They don't cause weight gain. Examples of these drugs are sitagliptin, saxagliptin, and linagliptin.

GLP-1 receptor agonists

These drugs slow digestion and help lower blood sugar levels. Their use is often associated with some weight loss. This class of medications isn't recommended for use by itself.

Exenatide and liraglutide are examples of GLP-1 receptor agonists. Possible side effects include nausea and an increased risk of pancreatitis.

Gliptins work by preventing the breakdown of a naturally occurring hormone called GLP-1. GLP-1 helps the body produce insulin in response to high blood glucose levels, but is rapidly broken down.

By preventing this breakdown, the gliptins (linagliptin, saxagliptin, sitagliptin and vildagliptin) prevent high blood glucose levels but don't result in episodes of hypoglycemia.

You may be prescribed a gliptin if you're unable to take sulphonylureas or glitazones, or in combination with them. They're not associated with weight gain.

SGLT2 inhibitors

These are the newest diabetes drugs on the market. They work by preventing the kidneys from reabsorbing sugar into the blood. Instead, the sugar is excreted in the urine.

Examples include canagliflozin and dapagliflozin. Side effects may include yeast infections and urinary tract infections, increased urination and hypotension.

Insulin therapy.

Some people who have type 2 diabetes need insulin therapy as well. In the past, insulin therapy was used as a last resort, but today it's often prescribed sooner because of its benefits.

Exenatide is a GLP-1 agonist, an injectable treatment that acts in a similar way to the natural hormone GLP-1.

It's injected twice a day and boosts insulin production when there are high blood glucose levels, reducing blood glucose without the risk of hypoglycemia episodes.

It also leads to modest weight loss in many people who take it. It's mainly used in people on metformin plus sulphonylureas, who are obese. A once-weekly product has also been introduced.

Another GLP-1 agonist called Liraglutide is a once-daily injection (Exenatide is given twice a day). Like Exenatide, Liraglutide is mainly used for people on metformin plus sulphonylureas, who are obese, and in clinical trials, it's been shown to cause modest weight loss.

Acarbose

Acarbose helps prevent your blood glucose level from increasing too much after you eat a meal. It slows down the rate at which your digestive system breaks carbohydrates down into glucose.

Acarbose isn't often used to treat type 2 diabetes because it usually causes side effects, such as bloating and diarrhea. However, it may be prescribed if you can't take other kinds of medicine for type 2 diabetes.

Nateglinide and repaglinide

Nateglinide and repaglinide stimulate the release of insulin by your pancreas. They're not commonly used, but may be an option if you have meals at irregular times. This is because their effects don't last very long, but they're effective when taken just before you eat.

Nateglinide and repaglinide can cause side effects, such as weight gain and hypoglycemia (low blood sugar).

If you have type 2 diabetes, your risk of developing heart disease, stroke and kidney disease is increased. To reduce your risk of developing other serious health conditions, you may be advised to take other medicines, including:

• Antihypertensive medications to control high blood pressure

• A statin, such as simvastatin or atorvastatin, to reduce high cholesterol

• Low-dose aspirin to prevent stroke

• An angiotensin-converting enzyme (ACE) inhibitor, such as enalapril, lisinopril or ramipril, if you have the early signs of diabetic kidney disease

Making lifestyle changes in type 2 diabetes.

If you're diagnosed with type 2 diabetes, you'll need to look after your health very carefully for the rest of your life.

After being diagnosed with type 2 diabetes, or if you're at risk of developing it, the first step is to look at your diet and lifestyle, and make any necessary changes.

Three major areas that you'll need to look closely at are your:

- Diet
- Weight
- Level of physical activity

By eating healthily, losing weight (if you're overweight) and exercising regularly, you may be able to keep your blood glucose in a safe and healthy level without the need for other types of treatment or drugs.

Diet

• Increasing the amount of fiber in your diet and reduce your fat intake, particularly saturated fat, can help prevent type 2 diabetes, as well as manage the condition if you already have it. You should:

• Increase your consumption of high-fiber foods, such as wholegrain bread and cereals, beans and lentils, and fruit and vegetables

• Choose foods that are low in fat – Replace butter, ghee and coconut oil with low-fat spreads and vegetable oil

• Choose skimmed and semi-skimmed milk, and low-fat yogurts

• Eat fish and lean meat rather than fatty or processed meat, such as sausages and burgers

- Grill, bake, poach or steam food instead of frying or roasting it

- Avoid high-fat foods, such as mayonnaise, chips, crisps, pastries, poppadums' and samosas

- Eat fruit, unsalted nuts and low-fat yogurts as snacks instead of cakes, biscuits, Bombay mix or crisps.

Weight

If you're overweight or obese (you have a body mass index (BMI) of 30 or over), you should lose weight. By gradually reducing your calorie intake and becoming more physically active you can lose weight.

Losing 5-10% of your overall body weight over the course of a year is a realistic initial target. You should aim to continue to lose weight until you've achieved and maintained a BMI within the healthy range, which is:

- $18.5\text{-}24.9\text{kg/m}^2$ for the general population
- $18.5\text{-}22.9\text{kg/m}^2$ for people of South Asian or Chinese origin ('South Asian' means Bangladesh, Bhutan, India, Indian-Caribbean, Maldives, Nepal, Pakistan and Sri Lanka)

If you have a BMI of 30kg/m^2 or more (27.5kg/m^2 or more for people of South Asian or Chinese origin), you need a structured weight loss program, which should form part of an intensive lifestyle change program.

To achieve changes in your diet, you should consult a dietician or a related healthcare professional for a personal assessment and tailored advice about diet and physical activity.

Physical activity

Being physically active is crucial in preventing or managing type 2 diabetes.

For adults who are 19-64 years of age, the physical activity guidelines are:

- 150 minutes (2 hours and 30 minutes) of "moderate-intensity" aerobic activity – such as cycling or fast walking – a week, which can be taken in sessions of 10 minutes or more, and muscle-strengthening activities on two or more days a week that work all major muscle groups (legs, hips, back, tummy (abdomen), chest, shoulders and arms)

An alternative recommendation is to do a minimum of:

- 75 minutes of "vigorous-intensity" aerobic activity, such as running or a game of tennis every week, and muscle-strengthening activities on two or more days a week that work all major muscle groups (legs, hips, back, abdomen, chest, shoulders and arms)

In cases where the high activity levels are unrealistic, even small increases in physical activity will be beneficial to your health and act as a basis for future improvements.

Reduce the amount of time spent watching television or sitting in front of a computer. Going for a daily walk – for example, during your lunch break – is a good way of introducing regular physical activity into your schedule.

If you're overweight or obese, you may need to be more physically active to help you lose weight and maintain weight loss.

Your doctor, diabetes care team or dietician can give you more information and advice about losing weight and becoming more physically active.

Goals of Type 2 Diabetes Treatment.

When you want to control your blood sugar for a healthy and active life, first you have to set individual goals. These goals will show your effort. According to these goals, you can modify your lifestyle and treatment plan.

- Target Fasting blood glucose 6mmol/l and 2 hours after meal 8 mmol/l
- Your Target HbA1c level is less than 7%.
- Target blood pressure is under 140 / 80 and Target LDL level is below 100.
- Target blood cholesterol 4 mmol/L and a Tryglicaroid 1.7 mmol/L.

What is an insulin pump?

An insulin pump is a small device. It gives insulin according to your need. From Insulin Pump insulin is given through as small, flexible, plastic pipe inserted in your body. The cannula or tube is changed every 3 to 4 days.

If needed, a patient can get a large dose. Just by pressing a switch.

Insulin pumps stop the need of injection every day, saves you the pain.

Insulin, what are the types of insulin?

Since its discovery in 1921. Insulin has become the most prescribed drug in history.

As a drug, Insulin is made from animals (cow, pig etc.) or Bacteria genetically engineered to produce insulin same as human insulin. Some manufactured insulin is modified to work better. Those modified insulins are called an insulin analog.

There are many types of insulin.

- Rapid Acting Insulin as the name implies, this type of insulin works within 15 min of injection and works up to 4 hours.
- Short-acting insulin or regular insulin starts working in 30 minutes. It continues to work up to 6 hours.
- Intermediate-acting Insulin - NPH gets into the blood in 2 hours. And works up to 18 hours.
- Long-acting insulin reaches blood in 3 or 4 hours after injection. And works up to 24 hours.

There is mixed insulin containing rapid acting insulin analog and medium or long acting insulin. Given before meals. They start to work 2 hours after injection.

What type of insulin do you need?

The kind of insulin you need must be advised by your doctor. It can be harmful if insulin is given in vein or muscle or large dose. Never change your treatment plan without consulting your doctor or health care professional.

In general, patients with Type 2 Diabetes needs multiple doses of insulin injection or continuous insulin infusion. Insulin is usually advised when blood glucose is not controlled with oral medicines.

To reduce the chance of hypoglycemia, insulin analogs should be used.

Insulin Dose Explained

The objective of injectable insulin is to duplicate the secretion of insulin by the normal pancreas. Regular insulin secretion from pancreas has two parts:

Basal insulin –

usually from a normal functioning pancreas, a small amount of insulin called the basal secretion of insulin circulates in the blood at all times. This can be duplicated in a patient with Type 2 Diabetes by taking long-acting insulin. The other way of getting a small amount of insulin continuously is with an insulin pump.

Basal insulin deals with the glucose produced by your liver. If you skip a meal, your basal insulin alone should be able to keep your blood glucose levels stable.

Bolus insulin –

normally the pancreas secretes a large amount of insulin at the time of meals, called the bolus secretion. This number is duplicated by taking rapid-acting insulin just before the meal or regular insulin 30 minutes before meals.

While basal insulin influences your blood glucose levels in between meals, it's the bolus (fast-acting) insulin that deals with the carbohydrate contained in any food and drink you have.

Insulin is manufactured in strengths of 100 units per milliliter. Your doctor will determine the dose of insulin consisting of a basal dose and a bolus dose. Usually, the insulin dose is calculated by Patient's weight in kilogram and multiplied by 0.3.

The first time a patient takes insulin, the dosage is based upon a calculated total daily dose. Your doctor will make this decision on dose,

Doctors usually follow these steps to calculate insulin dose:

- Multiply the weight of the patient in kilograms by 0.3. (for example, if a patients' weight is 40 kg, insulin needed (40 multiplied by 0.3) 12 unit per day.
- Divide the total daily dose into basal and bolus dose by simply dividing it in half. (for example, if a patient needs 12 units per day he should get a 6-unit basal dose and 6-unit bolus dose.
- The basal dose is taken once or sometimes split into two times a day, usually in the morning (two third of the full dose) and (remaining one third) at bedtime. It is best to divide the basal dose into a large number of units in the morning and a few units at bedtime.

Factors influencing the bolus dose of Insulin.

Your doctor will decide how much insulin you need. A Bolus dose of insulin is calculated using three primary factors.

The level of the blood glucose before a meal – if before meal blood glucose is high you need to add two units of insulin with your regular dose. If the premeal blood glucose is lower than ideal, you need to decrease two units of insulin from your daily dose.

The amount of carbohydrate in your meal – generally for every 15 grams of carbohydrate 1-unit insulin is added. But the amount of adjustment varies with different people at different ages.

Whether exercise has been or is about to be done - Exercise lowers the blood glucose. But sometimes exercise may increase blood glucose. Try to maintain a blood glucose of about 150 mg/dl during exercise. Take glucose in the form of three to four glucose tablets if the blood glucose falls below 100 mg/dl. Take rapid-acting insulin and wait to exercise if the blood glucose is over 300 mg/dl. Take half the usual dose before a meal before exercise if the blood glucose is satisfactory.

Try to exercise at the same time every day.

How to keep and store insulin?

Keep the insulin you are currently using at room temperature in a cool, dry place and away from direct light.

Best to keep it under 30 C. Cold insulin injection is painful. If you keep regular use insulin in a fridge be sure to take it out from fridge 30 minutes before using it. Keep it at room temperature for 30 min before giving the injection.

- Store insulin for an extended period of time at 4 to 6-degree temperature.
- Don't place insulin in, or close to, the freezer compartment.
- Never heat insulin or keep it beside the source of heat (oven, TV, locked car, radiator etc.)
- For travel use a special cold bag or use a flask.
- Check the expiration date and color of insulin. If there is clamps or the color changed do not use it.

Don't use insulin if:
- Clear insulin has turned cloudy or changed color
- The expiration date has been reached
- Insulin has been frozen solid or exposed to high temperatures
- Lumps or flakes can be seen inside the vial.
- The vial has been opened for more than 28 days.

Where to inject insulin?

Insulin is given just under the skin for a longer effect. And most of the time it's self-administered. It's easy to give insulin injection in your belly, back and thighs. But remember not to give insulin at the same site regularly. Rotate the sites every time.

Steps to give an insulin injection?

Your doctor will calculate how much insulin needed (Dose). Also, the doctor will tell you how many times insulins is necessary and type of insulin needed. Never change the dose or schedule without consulting your doctor first.

Follow these steps to give an insulin injection

- Wash your hand with soap and water.
- Check the insulin bottle for the expiration date.
- Check the insulin bottle for clamps, color change. If there is clamps or color change, do not give insulin from that vial.
- Wipe the cap of the insulin bottle with an alcohol pad.
- Clean the skin where you will get the injection with an alcohol pad or soap and water.
- Pinch skin and fat with the thumb.
- Push the needle into your skin: With your other hand, hold the syringe at a 45-degree angle. Make sure the needle is all the way into the skin.
- Let go of the pinched tissue before you inject the insulin
- Inject the insulin: Press the plunger with your thumb.
- Use slow and steady push until the insulin is gone.
- Wait for 5 to 10 seconds.
- Pull out the needle: Pull out the needle at the same angle you put it in. Press your injection site with cotton for a few seconds.

Use Insulin syringes only once. Throw away used needles and syringes in a hard container so that the needles cannot stick through. Close the container with a screw-on cap. Keep the container out of reach of children and pets.

How to decrease pain when giving insulin?

•   Inject insulin at room temperature. If insulin is stored in the fridge, remove it 30 minutes before you inject it. Cold insulin injection is painful.

•   Remove all air bubbles from the syringe before the injection.

•   If you clean your skin with an alcohol pad, wait until it has dried before you inject insulin.

•   Relax the muscles at the injection site.

•   Avoid changing the direction of the needle during insertion or removal.

•   Do not reuse disposable needles. Because needles get blunt and cause pain.

•   Try numbing the area of injection by use of an ice cube. Keep the ice cube pressed to skin for 2 minutes just before injection.

•   Always use a different site to give the injection.

What is the target blood glucose level?

As a general rule, target fasting blood glucose should be 4 to 7 mmol/L. And 2 hours after food blood glucose target is 9 mmol/L. Your doctor will advise and explain the target blood glucose level perfect for you.

Long-term Complications of Type 2 Diabetes?

Long-term complications from Type 2 diabetes can be easy to ignore, especially in the early stages when you're feeling fine. But diabetes affects many major organs, including your heart, blood vessels, nerves, eyes and kidneys. Controlling your blood sugar levels can help prevent these complications.

Long-term complications of diabetes develop gradually; they can eventually be disabling or even life-threatening. Some of the potential complications of diabetes include:

Heart and blood vessel disease.

Diabetes dramatically increases the risk of various cardiovascular problems, including coronary artery disease with chest pain (angina), heart attack, stroke, narrowing of arteries (atherosclerosis) and high blood pressure.

Nerve damage (neuropathy).

Excess sugar can injure the walls of the tiny blood vessels (capillaries) that nourish your nerves, especially in the legs. This nerve damage can cause tingling, numbness, burning or pain that usually begins at the tips of the toes or fingers and gradually spreads upward. Poorly controlled blood sugar can eventually cause you to lose all sense of feeling in the affected limbs. Damage to the nerves that control digestion can cause problems with nausea, vomiting, diarrhea or constipation. For men, erectile dysfunction may be an issue.

Kidney damage (nephropathy).

The kidneys contain millions of tiny blood vessel clusters that filter waste from your blood. Diabetes can damage this delicate filtering system. Severe damage can lead to kidney failure or irreversible end-stage kidney disease, which often eventually requires dialysis or a kidney transplant.

Eye damage.

Diabetes can damage the blood vessels of the retina (diabetic retinopathy), potentially leading to blindness. Diabetes also increases the risk of other serious vision conditions, such as cataracts and glaucoma.

Foot damage.

Nerve damage in the feet or poor blood flow to the feet increases the risk of various foot complications. Left untreated, cuts and blisters can become serious infections, which may heal poorly. Severe damage might require toe, foot or leg amputation.

Hearing impairment.

Hearing problems are more common in people with diabetes.

Skin conditions.

Diabetes may leave you more susceptible to skin problems, including bacterial and fungal infections.

Alzheimer's disease.

Type 2 diabetes may increase the risk of Alzheimer's disease. The poorer your blood sugar control, the greater the risk appears to be. The exact connection between these two conditions remains unclear.

Hyperosmolar Hyperglycemic Nonketotic Syndrome (HHNS)

Hyperosmolar Hyperglycemic Nonketotic Syndrome, or HHNS, is a serious condition most frequently seen in older persons. It is a short-term complication of diabetes. HHNS can happen to people with either type 1 or type 2 diabetes that is not being controlled correctly, but it occurs more often in people with type 2 diabetes. HHNS is usually brought on by something else, such as an illness or infection.

In HHNS, blood sugar levels rise, and your body try to get rid of the excess sugar by passing it into your urine. You make lots of urine at first, and you have to go to the bathroom more often. Later you may not have to go to the bathroom as often, and your urine becomes very dark. Also, you may be very thirsty. Even if you are not thirsty, you need to drink liquids. If you don't drink enough fluids at this point, you can get dehydrated.

If HHNS continues, the severe dehydration will lead to seizures, coma and eventually death. HHNS may take days or even weeks to develop. Know the warning signs of HHNS.

What are the Warning Signs of Hyperosmolar Hyperglycemic Nonketotic Syndrome?

Blood sugar level over 600 mg/dl

Dry, parched mouth

Extreme thirst (although this may gradually disappear)

Warm, dry skin that does not sweat

High fever (over 101 degrees Fahrenheit, for example)

Sleepiness or confusion

Loss of vision

Hallucinations (seeing or hearing things that are not there)

Weakness on one side of the body

If you have any of these symptoms, call someone on your health care team.

How to handle Hyperosmolar Hyperglycemic Nonketotic Syndrome

Hyperosmolar hyperglycemic nonketotic syndrome (HHNS) is rare, but you should be aware of it and know how to manage it. HHNS is when your blood glucose level goes way too high, and if you don't treat it, it can cause death.

HHNS is most likely to occur when you're sick, and older adults are most likely to develop it. It starts when your blood glucose level starts to climb: when that happens, your body will try to get rid of all the excess glucose through frequent urination. That dehydrates your body, and you'll become very thirsty.

Unfortunately, when you're sick, you can't always rehydrate your body as you should. You might have trouble keeping fluids down, for example. When you don't rehydrate your body, the blood glucose level continues to climb, and it can eventually go so high that it will send you into a coma.

To avoid hyperosmolar hyperglycemic nonketotic syndrome, you should keep a close watch on your blood glucose level when you're sick (always pay attention to your blood glucose level, but pay particular attention when sick).

Talk to your healthcare professional about having a sick-day plan to follow.

Macrovascular Complications of type 2 diabetes

Type 2 diabetes can also affect the large blood vessels, causing plaque to eventually build up and potentially leading to a heart attack, stroke or vessel blockage in the legs (peripheral vascular disease).

To prevent heart disease and stroke as a result of diabetes, you should manage your diabetes well, but you should also make heart-healthy choices in other areas of your life: don't smoke, keep your blood pressure under control, and pay attention to your cholesterol.

It is important to have your cholesterol checked annually. Your doctor should check your blood pressure every office visit. Also at every office visit, the doctor should check the pulse in your feet to make sure there is proper circulation.

Diabetic ketoacidosis or DKA?

DKA (Diabetic Ketoacidosis) is a dangerous short-term complication of Diabetes. In Type 2 Diabetes pancreas can't produce enough insulin for the need of the body. Without insulin, glucose can't enter & work in the cell. This extra Glucose accumulates in the blood, causing hyperglycemia.

Glucose is the primary source of energy for our body. To function our body needs glucose. When glucose is absent in cells to meet the energy demand of our body, stored fat of the body starts to breakdown. Breakdown of fat to supply the energy our body needs leads to ketone production. With ketone blood becomes acidic and diabetic ketoacidosis occurs.

DKA is a medical emergency and must be treated at a hospital.

What is the cause of DKA?

The cause of DKA includes Infection (Pneumonia or lung infection or Urine infection). Missed insulin injection, trauma, stroke or heart failure.

DKA is a medical emergency, and treatment can only be given at hospital/clinic. To confirm DKA a home urine test can be done, which will show dark purple color. In DKA blood sugar is high, more than 250mg/dl (13.8 mmol/L).

To prevent DKA, you should never miss insulin injection. Monitor signs of DKA, you should be able to recognize symptoms of DKA.

How to recognize DKA?

Fruity Smell of acetone is a major sign of diabetic ketoacidosis.

With fast & shallow breathing pattern.

Sweating with cold, clammy skin.

Increased thirst.

Abdominal pain, Nausea & vomiting.

Confusion or coma. These are symptoms of DKA (Diabetic Keto Acidosis).

Ketones: Testing at home

Checking Ketone in urine is the confirmatory test of Diabetic Keto Acidosis (DKA) Ketone is measured easily by putting a ketone strip into a tube containing urine.

If your blood glucose is above 250 mg/dl (13.8 mmol/L). Check urine for ketone.

To do the test, collect urine in a plastic cup and place a ketone strip in urine. The strip will change color. Compare the color with the color chart, and you get the result. There are four possible results, negative, low, medium or high.

High ketones with high blood glucose mean that you may be on the way to DKA (Diabetic ketoacidosis). You should contact your doctor or diabetes health team.

Hypoglycemia diagnosis, and treatment?

Hypoglycemia or low blood glucose is another short-term complication of Diabetes. It is a common but dangerous condition. The good thing is hypoglycemia shows certain symptoms. Which makes it easy to recognize by you.

Hypoglycemia symptoms start to show as soon as blood glucose level becomes 75 mg/dl (4.1 mmol/L) or lower. Symptoms include Anxiety, Irritability, Numbness in the lips, fingers, and toes.

The cause of hypoglycemia?

Most of the time accidentally taking insulin in high dose causes hypoglycemia. Another cause of hypoglycemia is taking the wrong type of insulin. Other causes are, having missed a meal or taking a small amount of food and too much physical exercise.

Some drugs may lower blood glucose leading to hypoglycemia. Such drugs are Beta-blockers for hypertension, Aspirin for a headache, etc.

Mild hypoglycemia is treated with a small portion of food. Give carbohydrate or sugar containing drinks.

Types of Hypoglycemia and treatment?

When the blood glucose level becomes 65mg/dl (3.6 mmol/L) or lower, it's called moderate hypoglycemia. Symptoms include Rapid heartbeat. The sensation of hunger. Sweating and Whiteness or pallor of the skin.

Moderate hypoglycemia needs 4 to 5 glucose tablets or oral glucose. Recheck blood glucose after 20 minutes. If the blood glucose level is still low, give more glucose tablet or powder and recheck again.

When blood glucose level is less than 55 mg/dl (3.05 mmol/L), it's called severe hypoglycemia. Symptoms include Confusion and trouble concentrating, Convulsions, Dizziness, Fatigue, Feeling of warmth, headache, Reduced consciousness or coma, and Slurred speech.

Severe hypoglycemia is a medical emergency. You must take the patient to the hospital as soon as possible. Use a glucagon injection if prescribed by your doctor and available.

There are some common things you can do in any hypoglycemia or low blood glucose. If the patient is conscious and can take food by mouth. He should be given 3 to 4 glucose tablets or 15 grams of glucose powder with a half glass of water or you can give 15ml or three teaspoons of honey. Recheck blood glucose 20 minutes. If the blood glucose level is still low, you can give more glucose tablet or honey.

If the patient is unconscious or unable to take food. Consult your doctor or health care provider.

Instead of glucose tablet (if unavailable). You can give sugar containing drinks such as Apple or orange juice.

Glucagon injection for hypoglycemia?
Glucagon is a hormone, and it's given in severe hypoglycemia to protect the body.

Glucagon comes in a package containing powder glucagon and water for injection in 2 vials. A syringe with needle is also available. Check the expiration date of glucagon injection.

First, take water from a vial with syringe. Inject the water in the powder containing bottle. Shake to mix powder glucagon with water. Take mixed drug using the syringe and inject into muscle. In hip or upper arm.

Patient and family members should learn the symptoms of hypoglycemia. And how to give a glucagon injection.

You need to have glucagon injection, glucose monitoring device and sugar tablet with you at all time.

What happens in hyperglycemia?

Hyperglycemia means height level of glucose in the blood. It happens when we miss the treatment. Eat plenty sugar containing food or drinks. Stress or any infection also increases blood glucose.

Excessive blood glucose damage organs such as heart, blood vessels, eyes, nerves, etc. of the body.

High blood glucose affects the body slowly; it causes;

Eye disease -cataract and retinopathy.

Kidney disease - damage the kidneys.

Nervous system damage.

Heart disease.

Diabetic neuropathy

All patients should be screened by a doctor for diabetic peripheral neuropathy (DPN) once every year. Symptoms of diabetic neuropathy would be numbness, tingling or burning sensation of hands & foot.

To prevent diabetic neuropathy strictly keep blood glucose at ideal levels. Tight control of blood sugar is the only option.

Managing Diabetic neuropathy and its complications?

Diabetic neuropathy — a type of nerve damage that can occur over time due to high blood sugar in those who have diabetes. It is a common but serious complication of diabetes. In addition to the pain that diabetic neuropathy can cause, it can also lead to other complications, such as problems with your digestive system, urinary tract, blood vessels and heart.

Specific treatments exist for many of the complications of diabetic neuropathy, including:

Urinary tract problems. Antispasmodic medications (anticholinergics), behavioral techniques such as timed urination, and devices such as pessaries. Pessaries are rings which can be inserted into the vagina to prevent urine leakage — may be helpful in treating loss of bladder control. A combination of therapies may be more efficient.

Digestive problems. Gastroparesis is a condition in which the stomach empties too slowly or not at all. You can usually prevent gastroparesis by eating smaller, more-frequent meals, reducing fiber and fat in the diet, and, for many people, eating soups and pureed foods. Diarrhea, constipation, and nausea may be helped with dietary changes, probiotics and medications.

Low blood pressure on standing (orthostatic hypotension). This is often helped with simple lifestyle measures, such as avoiding alcohol, drinking plenty of water and standing up slowly. Your doctor may recommend an abdominal binder, a compression support for your abdomen, and compression stockings. Several medications, either alone or together, also may be used to treat orthostatic hypotension.

Sexual dysfunction. Sildenafil (Revatio, Viagra), tadalafil (Adcirca, Cialis) and vardenafil (Levitra, Staxyn) can improve sexual function in some men, but these medications aren't effective or safe for everyone. When drugs don't work, many people turn to vacuum devices, or, if these fail, to penile implants. Women may be helped with vaginal lubricants.

For some people, these symptoms are mild; for others, diabetic neuropathy can be painful, disabling and even fatal. Work with your doctor to determine the best approach to managing your diabetic neuropathy complications.

Diabetic Retinopathy

This is one of the major long-term complication of Type 2 Diabetes.

To prevent diabetic retinopathy or eye disease, you must control blood glucose level. Optimize glucose control will reduce the risk or slow the progression of retinopathy.

Diabetic Nephropathy

Uncontrolled blood glucose for a long time or in the case of patients with long-standing Diabetes causes kidney disease. It is called Diabetic Nephropathy. In Diabetic nephropathy, your kidneys slowly become nonfunctional.

Preventing Diabetic Nephropathy

To avoid diabetic kidney disease, you must control your blood glucose. Optimize glucose control will reduce the risk or slow the progression of diabetic kidney disease.

You have to control blood pressure. Keep the blood pressure close to a normal range such as 120 / 80 mmHg.

Control fat in the blood. Keep fat level (LDL or HDL) within normal range.

Treat urinary infection if you have a urinary infection.

Screening for Diabetic Nephropathy?

At least every year you should get your urine checked for urinary albumin and estimated glomerular filtration rate (eGFR)

Diet for Diabetic Nephropathy patients.

For people with diabetic kidney disease, reducing the amount of protein in the diet is essential.

Skin diseases in Type 2 Diabetes

Many skin conditions are unique to diabetes because of the treatment and complications of the disease. The most common and significant skin complications are:

• Bruises occur because insulin needles cut blood vessels.

• Vitiligo (loss of skin pigmentation) is part of the autoimmune aspect of type 1 diabetes and can't be prevented.

• Necrobiosis lipoidica, which also affects people without diabetes, creates patches of reddish-brown skin on the shins or ankles, and the skin becomes thin and ulcerated. Females tend to have this condition more often than males. Steroid injections are used to treat this condition, and the areas eventually become depressed and brown.

• Xanthelasma, which are small, yellow, flat areas called plaques on the eyelids, occur in Type 2 Diabetes even when cholesterol isn't elevated. Treatment may not be necessary.

• Alopecia, or loss of hair, occurs in people with diabetes, but the cause is unknown.

• Insulin hypertrophy is the accumulation of fatty tissue where insulin is injected. This condition is prevented by changing the injection site regularly.

• Insulin lipoatrophy is the loss of fat where the insulin is injected. Although the cause is unknown, this condition is rarely seen now that human insulin has replaced beef and pork insulin in diabetes treatment.

Diabetic thick skin is thicker than normal skin, occurs in people who have had diabetes for more than ten years.

Steps for Reducing complications of diabetes.

• Manage diabetes. Keep your blood glucose, blood pressure, and cholesterol at target levels.

• Regularly test your blood glucose level.

• See your doctor for all your recommended screening tests.

• Take your prescribed medicine regularly.

• Quit smoking.

• Exercise at least 30 min every alternate day.

• Follow a diet plan. Consult a dietitian for specific diet plan for you.

• Limit alcohol intake.

• Maintain an ideal weight.

Ideal body weight for Type 2 Diabetes?

Managing and keeping ideal weight is essential for any diabetic patient. Balanced weight lowers the chance of heart and kidney disease.

To understand ideal body weight, we have to know Body Mass Index or BMI. It's calculated by dividing your weight in Kilograms by your height in meter squared. A BMI below 18.5 is underweight. A BMI from 18.5 to 24.99 is the ideal weight. BMI 30 or more is obese.

Try to keep your BMI in the normal range. If your BMI is high, try to lose 5 -10% of your body weight. Be sure to consult with your doctor and approach the weight loss gradually. Remember, you should not start any weight loss program or diet without consulting your doctor.

Sometimes diabetic patients tend to be underweight and malnourished. The underweight body makes it difficult to stay healthy. Consult your dietitian how to gain weight. Some weight gain tips are, eat small but frequent meals. Add more fat (margarine, cheese, butter, oil, etc.) to your diet. Eat dried fruit and nuts.

Improve blood sugar levels after meals without using drugs

You can also improve blood sugar levels after meals without using drugs. There are two relevant approaches.

Take a small protein rich snack at early morning before breakfast, then after 2 hours take regular breakfast. This will reduce your blood glucose level by half. This is called the second meal effect, and although it has been recognized in non-diabetic individuals for almost a century, it has only recently been shown to work in people with type 2 diabetes.

Secondly, if you go out for a half hour walk after a meal (or do any physical activity), then the rise in blood glucose will be very much less compared to just sitting in a chair. This is because muscle tissue takes up glucose more rapidly during exercise, and the meal time rise in glucose is blunted.

Food for Type 2 Diabetes?

Food is a major component in the treatment of Type 2 Diabetes. Consulting with a dietitian for a personalized diet plan is important.

Bread, rice, potatoes, pasta & other starchy foods are the sources of carbohydrate. Carbohydrate is broken down to simple sugar in our body. It gives us all the energy we need. But Carbohydrate is also the primary source of glucose in the blood. We should watch how much carbohydrate we take with each meal. 40 to 60 percent of calories of our diet should come from carbohydrate.

Meat, fish, eggs, beans are sources of protein. Protein is needed for repair and growth of our body. Proteins do not have a direct effect on blood glucose. Protein is the main component of hormones, enzymes and antibodies. 10 to 20 percent of calories of our diet should come from protein. As part of a mixed meal, protein will slow the absorption of carbohydrate. Which is good for you.

Milk & dairy foods have essential vitamins and minerals. These products also have an effect on blood glucose.

Fruit & vegetables They contain essential vitamins. For a healthy diet fruit and vegetables are essential.

Goals of Nutrition Therapy for Adults with Diabetes

Goal one- Get a healthy and nutritious meal. Your food choice will help you achieve your desired blood glucose level, ideal body weight, target blood pressure. Your food choice will help you to prevent complications of diabetes.

Goal two – maintain the pleasure of eating. With Type 2 Diabetes there is a restriction on how much you eat. There is no restriction on what you eat. A good nutrition therapy should restore the pleasure of eating.

Goal three – a nutrition therapy will provide the individual with diabetes practical tools for day-to-day meal planning.

Tips on food.

Food is an essential part of Type 2 Diabetes treatment. It's best to consult with a dietitian to get your personalized diet plan. There are some common tips to help you with your diet.

• Eat more whole grains, fruits, & veggies. Limit or avoid foods that are high in fat, sugar, and white flour.

• Always use low-fat milk, cheese, yogurt and dairy products.

• Use pulses such as peas, beans or lentils to replace or reduce meat.

• Cut and remove visible fat from meat, from poultry product remove skin.

• When cooking, try to drain excess fat from meat before adding spices.

• Try to grill or baking instead of frying. Learn low-fat cooking methods.

• Eat carbohydrate that is slow to absorb with low glycemic Index.

• Eat pasta, basmati or easy cook rice, grainy bread such as granary, pumpernickel, rye, new potatoes, sweet potato, yam porridge, oats and natural muesli. These foods have a low glycemic index so that blood glucose will be low.

• For fat Choose unsaturated fats or oils, such as olive, rapeseed and sunflower oil. This fat will help you to lose weight. You can reach your target cholesterol level with low-fat diet.

• Use less butter, margarine and cheese.

• Eat fish at least once every week.

• Eat one portion of fruit such as 1 apple or banana or any other fruit you like every day.

• Avoid sugary drinks or smoothies.

• Do not take more than 6g of salt per day. Less salt reduces blood pressure and heart disease.

• Do not take alcohol more than 3 units per day. Half a pint of lager, ale, bitter or cider has 1-1½ units. Do not take alcohol on an empty stomach.

Tips on carbohydrate.

Eat carbohydrate (rice, pasta, etc.) in large chunks. It takes time to break down a large piece of carbohydrate inside our gut. So glucose is absorbed slowly, and blood glucose rises slowly.

Eat carbohydrate with fat to slow down absorption.

For the rapid rise of blood glucose (in the case of hypoglycemia) drink fruit juice or any beverage with food. Avoid fruit juice or any beverage if you are diabetic with high blood glucose.

Small snacks in between meals keep your blood glucose at a consistent level which is good for you.

Glycemic Index: What is it?

The glycemic index is a system of giving a number to every carbohydrate-containing food according to how much each food increases blood sugar. The glycemic index itself is not a diet plan, but one of the various tools — such as calorie counting or carbohydrate counting — for guiding food choices.

Many modern commercial diets, diet books and diet websites are based on the glycemic index, including the Zone Diet, Sugar Busters and the Slow-Carb Diet.

The purpose of a glycemic index (GI) diet is to eat carbohydrate-containing foods that are less likely to cause significant increases in blood sugar levels. The diet is a means to lose weight and prevent chronic diseases related to obesity such as diabetes and cardiovascular disease.

You might choose to follow the GI diet because you:

- Want to lose weight or maintain a healthy weight
- Need help planning and eating healthier meals
- Need help maintaining blood sugar levels as part of a diabetes treatment plan

The GI principle was first developed as a strategy for guiding food choices for people with diabetes. An international GI database is maintained by Sydney University Glycemic Index Research Services in Sydney, Australia. The database contains the results of studies conducted there and at other research facilities around the world.

A basic overview of carbohydrates, blood sugar, and GI values is helpful for understanding glycemic index diets.

Carbohydrates

Carbohydrates, or carbs, are a type of nutrient in foods. The three basic forms are sugars, starches and fiber. When you eat or drink something with carbs, your body breaks down the sugars and starches into a type of sugar called glucose, the primary source of energy for cells in your body. Fiber passes through your body undigested.

Two main hormones from your pancreas help regulate glucose in your bloodstream. The hormone insulin moves glucose from your blood into your cells. The hormone glucagon helps release glucose stored in your liver when your blood sugar (blood glucose) level is low. This process helps keep your body fueled and ensures a natural balance in blood glucose.

Different types of carbohydrates have properties that affect how quickly your body digests them and how quickly glucose enters your bloodstream.

Understanding GI values

There are various research methods for assigning a GI value to food. In general, the number is based on how much a food item raises blood glucose levels in healthy study participants compared with how much pure glucose raises their blood glucose. GI values are divided into three categories:

- Low GI: 1 to 55

- Medium GI: 56 to 69

- High GI: 70 and higher

For example, raw carrots have a GI value of 35. This means that if you eat carrots in a quantity that supplies 1.8 ounces or 50g carbohydrate your blood glucose level will be 35 percent of the blood glucose level after eating 1.8 ounces (50 grams) of pure glucose. It's confusing, I know. But easy when you know that high GI value means more glucose and usually bad for you.

Comparing GI values can help us to make healthier food choices. For example, an English muffin made with white wheat flour has a GI value of 77. A whole-wheat English muffin has a GI value of 45.

Limitations of GI values

One limitation of GI values is that they don't inform the quantity you would eat a particular food.

For example, watermelon has a GI value of 80, which would put it in the category of food to avoid. But watermelon has relatively few digestible carbohydrates in a typical serving. In other words, you have to eat a lot of watermelons to consume the standard test level of 1.8 ounces (50 grams) of digestible carbohydrates.

A GI value tells us nothing about other nutritional information. For example, whole milk has a GI value of 31 and a GL value of 4 for a 1-cup (250-milliliter) serving. But because of its high-fat content, whole milk is a poor choice for weight loss or weight control.

The published GI database is not an exhaustive list of foods, but a list of those foods that have been studied. Many healthy foods with low GI values are not in the database.

The GI value of any food item is affected by several factors, including how the food is prepared, how it is processed and what other foods are eaten at the same time.

What is Glycemic Load (GL)

Limitation of GI values is that they don't inform the quantity you would eat a particular food.

To address this problem, researchers have developed the idea of glycemic load (GL), a numerical value that indicates the change in blood glucose levels when you eat a typical serving of the food. For example, a 4.2-ounce (120-gram) serving of watermelon has a GL value of 5, which would identify it as a healthy food choice. For comparison, a 2. 8-ounce (80-gram) serving of raw carrots has a GL value of 2.

Sydney University's table of GI values also includes GL values. The values are grouped in the following manner:

- Low GL: 1 to 10

- Medium GL: 11 to 19

- High GL: 20 or more

Low GI Diet examples

A GI diet prescribes meals primarily of foods that have low values. Examples of foods with low, middle and high GI values include the following:

Low GI: Green vegetables, most fruits, raw carrots, kidney beans, chickpeas, lentils and bran breakfast cereals

Medium GI: Sweet corn, bananas, raw pineapple, raisins, oat breakfast cereals, and multigrain, oat bran or rye bread

High: White rice, white bread and potatoes

Commercial GI diets may describe foods as having slow carbs or fast carbs. In general, foods with a low GI value are digested and absorbed relatively slowly, and those with high values are absorbed quickly.

Commercial GI diets have different recommendations for portion size, as well as protein and fat consumption.

Benefit of GI diet

Studies of the benefits of GI diets have produced mixed results.

Weight loss

In a 2013 review of 23 published clinical trials of low-GI or low-GL diets, researchers concluded that the diets were "as effective as other dietary alternatives in inducing weight loss." In four of the studies, low-GI or low-GL diets resulted in statistically significant improvements in weight loss when compared with other diets. Ten studies showed a slight improvement — but not a statistically significant increase — in weight loss.

In another 2013 review, researchers analyzed clinical trials that compared two or more specialty diets to various dietary guidelines, including those published by the American Diabetes Association and the European Association for the Study of Diabetes. The results showed that low-carbohydrate diets and Mediterranean diets provided more weight-loss benefit than low-GI foods. (A Mediterranean diet includes olive oil, legumes, whole-grain cereals, fruit, vegetables, and modest amounts of meat and dairy products.)

A large trial published in 2010 followed 773 participants who had lost weight on a low-calorie diet. During the six months following this weight loss, people who ate a low-GI, high-protein diet were more likely to stick with their diet plan and not regain the weight they had lost.

Blood glucose control

A treatment goal for people with diabetes is to keep after eating and average blood glucose levels as close to nondiabetic levels as possible. This tight control helps prevent or slow the development of complications associated with the disease.

Some clinical studies have shown that a low-GI diet may help people with diabetes control blood glucose levels, although the observed effects may also be attributed to Low-calorie, high-fiber content of the diets prescribed in the study.

Cholesterol

Reviews of trials measuring the impact of low-GI index diets on cholesterol have shown fairly consistent evidence that such diets may help lower total cholesterol, as well as low-density lipoproteins (the "bad" cholesterol) — especially when a low-GI diet is combined with an increase in dietary fiber.

Appetite control

One theory about the effect of a low-GI diet is appetite control. The thinking is that high-GI food causes a rapid increase in blood glucose, a quick insulin response and a subsequent rapid return to feeling hungry. Low-GI foods would, in turn, delay feelings of hunger. Clinical investigations of this theory have produced mixed results.

Also, if a low-GI diet suppresses appetite, the long-term effect should be that such a diet would result over the long term in people choosing to eat less and better manage their weight. The long-term clinical research does not, however, demonstrate this effect.

The bottom line

For you to maintain your current weight, you need to burn as many calories as you consume. To lose weight, you need to burn more calories than you consume. Weight loss is best done with a combination of reducing calories in your diet and increasing your physical activity and exercise.

Selecting foods based on a glycemic index or glycemic load value may help you manage your weight because many foods that should be included in a well-balanced, low-fat, healthy diet with minimally processed foods — whole-grain products, fruits, vegetables and low-fat dairy products — have low GI values.

For some people, a commercial low-GI diet may provide necessary direction to help them make better choices for a healthy eating plan. The researchers who maintain the GI database caution, however, that the "glycemic index should not be used in isolation" and that other nutritional factors — calories, fat, fiber, vitamins and other nutrients — should be considered.

Physical Activity for Type 2 Diabetes.

Adults with Type 2 Diabetes should engage in physical activity such as aerobic exercise every alternate day. Gradually increase the amount of physical activity that you do each day until you reach 30-60 minutes of continuous activity.

To stay healthy, adults aged 19-64 should try to be active daily and should do:

At least 150 minutes of moderate aerobic activity such as cycling or fast walking every week, and strength exercises on two or more days a week that work all the major muscles (legs, hips, back, abdomen, chest, shoulders and arms).

75 minutes of vigorous aerobic activity, such as running or a game of singles tennis every week, and strength exercises on two or more days a week that work all the major muscles (legs, hips, back, abdomen, chest, shoulders and arms).

A mix of moderate and vigorous aerobic activity every week. For example, two 30-minute runs plus 30 minutes of fast walking equates to 150 minutes of moderate aerobic activity, and strength exercises on two or more days a week that work all the major muscles (legs, hips, back, abdomen, chest, shoulders and arms).

A rule of thumb is that one minute of vigorous activity provides the same health benefits as two minutes of moderate activity.

One way to do your recommended 150 minutes of weekly physical activity is to do 30 minutes on 5 days a week.

You should get up and walk for a brief time when you are inactive or desk bound for more than 90 min. Time spent in sedentary styles such as TV, computer or mobile games should be broken into small segments of less than 90 min. Do little physical activity during a commercial break in case of watching TV. During a game on the computer or mobile or tab take small breaks after each level.

Bariatric surgery a Radical Treatment for type 2 diabetes with obesity.

Surgery is an extreme choice to control your diabetes and weight. If you have type 2 diabetes and your body mass index (BMI) is greater than 35, you may be a candidate for weight-loss surgery (Bariatric surgery). Blood sugar levels return to normal in 55 to 95 percent of people with diabetes, depending on the procedure performed. Surgeries that bypass a portion of the small intestine have more of an effect on blood sugar levels than do other weight-loss surgeries.

Drawbacks to the surgery include its high cost, and there are risks involved, including a risk of death. Additionally, drastic lifestyle changes are required and long-term complications may include nutritional deficiencies and osteoporosis.

Pregnancy and type 2 diabetes.

Women with type 2 diabetes may need to alter their treatment during pregnancy. Many women will require insulin therapy during pregnancy. Cholesterol-lowering medications and some blood pressure drugs can't be used during pregnancy.

If you have signs of diabetic retinopathy, it may worsen during pregnancy. Visit your ophthalmologist during the first trimester of your pregnancy and at one year postpartum.

You may take a look at my book Pregnancy & Diabetes: Smallest Book with Everything You Need to Know

The book gives you a complete picture on GDM (Gestational Diabetes mellitus). It also provides information on pregnancy with type 1 or type 2 diabetes. If you are a pregnant mother with or without diabetes, this book gives all the information you need to protect you and your baby from the complications of GDM or other types of Diabetes.

Weight loss to achieve ideal body weight in type 2 diabetes.

Losing 5-10% of your overall body weight over the course of a year is a realistic initial target. You should aim to continue to lose weight until you've achieved and maintained a BMI within the healthy range, which is:

- 18.5-24.9kg/m^2 for the general population

- 18.5-22.9kg/m^2 for people of South Asian or Chinese origin ('South Asian' means Bangladesh, Bhutan, India, Indian-Caribbean, Maldives, Nepal, Pakistan and Sri Lanka)

If you have a BMI of 30kg/m² or more (27.5kg/m² or more for people of South Asian or Chinese origin), you need a structured weight loss program. You must start an intensive lifestyle change program.

Visiting your doctor?

You should visit a doctor or diabetes health team every six months' even if there are no physical complications. If any complication occurs, you must consult your doctor immediately.

Your doctor will check blood pressure on every visit. The target blood pressure is lower than 130/80 mmHg.

The doctor will check your foot for damage or ulcers (vascular damage).

Your doctor will check the eyes for injuries caused by Diabetes (Diabetic retinopathy). Every 2 years he will check and take a picture of the retina with a device called fundoscopy.

He will check your urine and run some blood test to see the condition of your kidneys (Diabetic Nephropathy).

He would check your nervous system for numbness in hands and legs (Diabetic Neuropathy).

These are painless physical exams done by your doctor or diabetes health team from time to time. It helps in early diagnosis if you have any complications of diabetes.

Type 2 diabetic patients' checkup every six months' even if there are no specific complaints.

Every six months Check:

- Blood pressure
- Weight
- Body mass index
- Waist circumference
- Foot care

Every year check:

- HbA1c
- Total cholesterol, LDL cholesterol and triglycerides
- Kidney check (urine microalbumin test)
- Medication review
- Smoking status
- Healthy eating plan
- Physical activity
- Self-care education

At least every two years:

- Eye examination (more frequently if evidence of disease)

Please note that the recommendations may be different in your country. It may be different for children or young adults.

Some myths about Diabetes

There is a common myth that diabetic patients can't have sugar or chocolate. Diabetes patients can have sugar or chocolate but have to adjust the insulin dose to control the extra sugar. Or workout a bit to burn the extra sugar if you are not on insulin.

It's best to avoid sugar and sugar-containing foods as much as possible.

Another myth is diabetic people can't play sports. It's also a misconception. A well-controlled Diabetic can play sports and do physical Exercise. It's even good for him. But he should be careful with low blood glucose (hypoglycemia) and keep glucometer and some glucose tablet and glucagon kit handy.

Smoking and Type 2 Diabetes

Smoking is a significant health hazard even without diabetes. With diabetes, smoking creates many complications. You already know what the harmful effects of smoking are. You have to quit smoking, and there is no other option.

Following are the benefits of quitting smoking.

•   Only 20 minutes after quitting your heart rate and blood pressure improve.

•   In 8-hour nicotine is out of your body, the oxygen level in your blood improves. With oxygen, you feel stronger and healthier.

- In 48 hours of quitting your sense of smell and taste improve dramatically.

- In a month, you become healthier with reduced chance of heart attack and stroke.

- In three months your breathing improves. A chronic cough and cold are reduced just in 3 months after quitting.

- In 6 months your skin will improve. You will look younger and feel younger.

Immunization for Type 2 Diabetes patient

Take all routine vaccinations;

You should get an Influenza vaccination every year.

You should get Pneumococcal polysaccharide vaccine 23 or PPSV23 vaccine.

Adults 65 or more years of age, should get Pneumococcal conjugate vaccine 13 (PCV13), followed by PPSV23, 6–12 months after initial vaccination. If not previously vaccinated.

Get hepatitis B vaccination.

Maintaining a Quality Life with Type 2 Diabetes.

To have a quality life and manage it with Type 2 Diabetes you have to control your blood glucose level, blood pressure and blood cholesterol level.

The keys to the maintenance of a high quality of life with Type 2 Diabetes Are

Regular measuring of blood glucose and knowing how to respond to high and low blood glucose.

Get regular examination (6 months or yearly) by your doctor or healthcare professional.

Learn how to count carbohydrate quantity in meals and adjust insulin dose accordingly.

Enjoying good food that's also nutritious.

Exercise regularly to keep your muscles in excellent shape This will help to keep your metabolism functioning well.

Get sufficient sleep at least 8 hours every day.

Avoiding blaming yourself when things don't go exactly as you planned.

Living with Type 2 Diabetes.

There are few things you can do to improve your life with Type 2 Diabetes.

Maintain a balance between control and freedom. Do not try to control every high blood glucose. It will stress you out. Focus on overall correction of blood glucose.

Anger with Type 2 Diabetes is a natural response. We become angry with all the limitations due to Type 2 Diabetes. Talk to your friend or family. Try to find out the particular cause of anger. Sometimes you should get some freedom from a strict routine lifestyle.

Be aware that you should never blame yourself for the fact that you have diabetes. Type 2 Diabetes doesn't result from consuming too much sugar, failing to exercise sufficiently, or any other failure that you may imagine.

Don't overreact to any temporary loss of control or increased glucose level. Try to find the cause. Control of the blood glucose may be lost temporarily when you get sick with a virus or other problems. When it happens, move on and try to restore the control as soon as possible.

Recognize that depression can occur in patients with Type 2 Diabetes. If your sleep is disturbed, if you don't feel like eating, if your general positive outlook changes to sadness and unhappiness, it may be the time to consult your doctor.

Future of Type 2 Diabetes

We now know that the problem in type 2 diabetes relates to high-fat levels in the pancreas and the liver. When calorie intake is sharply decreased - either by a diet or by weight loss surgery - the fat levels in these organs drop and it has been shown that the function of the pancreas and liver returns to normal.

A single injection each week, which could help the body respond more appropriately to food, and at the same time would help with weight control. It is the future of type 2 diabetes treatment. This is what GLP-1 agonists do. These drugs, which mimic a naturally occurring gut hormone, that tell the body to produce more insulin and the brain to stop eating. These are already available, and a long-acting injection is well on its way.

Conclusion

Thank you for reading this book. I wish you a safe, healthy and fulfilling life with diabetes. If a single patient is helped through this book and information that is the biggest success of this book. The biggest success of me.

I humbly request you, please write a small review (1 or 2 lines) of this book.

Share the link with your friends, family or coworkers, if you think this book can help with their diabetes. Of course, sharing the link is beneficial for me but it also helps diabetic patients find this book. So please share it to help diabetic patients worldwide.

Wishing you a happy and prolonged like

THE END

About Author

Dr. Shahriar Mostafa earned his MBBS degree in 2009. Then completed his Master's degree in Public Health in 2013. He works in at a Medical College Hospital for last seven years. He wants to write simple, easy to read and small patient education books to reach a larger audience.

Other Book by Dr. Shahriar

Pregnancy & Diabetes: Smallest Book with Everything You Need to Know

This book gives you a complete picture on GDM (Gestational Diabetes mellitus). It also provides information on pregnancy with type 1 or type 2 diabetes. If you are a pregnant mother with or without diabetes, this book gives all the information you need to protect you and your baby from the complications of GDM or other types of Diabetes.

Type 1 diabetes: Smallest Book with Everything You Need to Know.

You can finish this book in just 1 hour. In just 1 hour you will have all relevant information on Type one diabetes. This book will give the confidence, hope, and knowledge to live a normal happy life with Type One Diabetes.

High Blood Pressure: Control with and without Medicine
Hundreds of people with Hypertension are changing their condition. They are taking charge of their treatment for high blood pressure.

In this book, you will find all these answers you need to know about high blood pressure. Here I have given pro and cons of drug and non-drug (Herbal, Homeopathic, Meditation) treatments proven to be useful for hypertension. Also, included and explained treatments that are useless for hypertension.

I hope after reading this book you can choose a plan to control and prevent hypertension. You can choose a plan that works for you.

www.ingramcontent.com/pod-product-compliance
Lightning Source LLC
Chambersburg PA
CBHW022345290526
45786CB00014B/2483